CATARRH

A Thorough Examination of the Signs and Causes of Catarrh Prevention

CARL JUAN

Table of Contents

Introductory

Overproduction of mucus or inflammation of the respiratory or mucous membranes, most commonly the nose and throat, is commonly referred to as catarrh. Typical signs include a sore throat, a tickle at the back of the nose, and a cough. Infections (like the common cold), allergies, and irritants are only some of the potential reasons of catarrh. The formation of thick, dark mucus is a typical sign of many respiratory disorders. Rest, fluids, and over-the-counter or prescribed drugs to alleviate symptoms are common approaches to treating catarrh, although treating the underlying cause is preferable.

CHAPTER ONE
Various Catarrh Causes

Excessive mucus production or inflammation of the mucous membranes, most commonly in the respiratory system, is referred to as catarrh. Catarrh isn't often subdivided into subtypes, but the symptoms might vary widely depending on what's triggering the inflammation and where it's taking place in the body. The following are examples of catarrh subtypes:

- **Nasal Catarrh:** This type of catarrh primarily affects the nasal passages, resulting in symptoms such as a runny or stuffy nose. It is commonly accompanied with illnesses like the common cold, allergic rhinitis, or sinusitis.

• Throat catarrh is characterized by inflammation and an overabundance of mucus production in the throat, which can result in symptoms such as a painful throat, coughing, and a lump in the throat. Infections, postnasal drip, and irritants are all potential triggers.

• Inflammation and mucus production in the bronchial tubes (airways leading to the lungs) characterize bronchial catarrh. Bronchitis and chronic obstructive pulmonary disease (COPD) are common causes of this catarrh.

• Catarrh of the ear occurs when the Eustachian tubes, which go from the middle ear to the base of the throat, become clogged with mucus or inflamed. Pain, fullness, and sometimes difficulty hearing are all symptoms of this illness. It's often linked to a cold or the flu.

• Inflammation and mucus production in the sinuses (tiny air-filled chambers in the skull) are the hallmarks of sinus catarrh. Sinus pressure, headaches, and facial pain are all possible outcomes. Sinusitis and other similar conditions may induce sinus catarrh.

These manifestations of catarrhal symptoms in various regions of the respiratory system are described, but they are not separate medical disorders. A healthcare provider should diagnose and treat the underlying cause of catarrh, which could be an infection, allergy, irritant, or persistent illness. The catarrh and the underlying cause may dictate the treatment strategy.

Factors That Set It Off

The appropriate treatment for catarrh typically depends on what caused or prompted it. Catarrh typically results from the following causes and triggers:

• **Infections:** Viruses and bacteria are typical culprits in causing catarrh. Allergies, the flu, sinus infections, bronchitis, and pneumonia are all respiratory illnesses. Infections cause irritation of the airways, leading to more mucus being produced.

• Catarrh can be brought on by an allergic reaction to pollen, dust, mold, pet dander, or another allergen. Symptoms of this catarrh include a runny or stuffy nose, sneezing, and throat irritation, and are sometimes linked to allergic rhinitis or hay fever.

• **Irritants:** Cigarette smoking, air pollution, strong scents, and chemicals are all known catarrh triggers. The irritation caused by these substances can lead to respiratory tract inflammation and an increase in mucus production.

• Throat irritation, catarrh, and coughing can be symptoms of GERD, a digestive illness in which acid from the stomach rushes back into the esophagus.

- Catarrh can be caused by a chronic ailment and can be persistent or recurrent. Bronchial catarrh with continuous mucus production and cough, for instance, is a common complication of COPD and chronic bronchitis.

- Postnasal drip occurs when mucus drips down the back of the throat as a result of excessive mucus production in the nasal passages. Catarrh of the throat and coughing may develop from infections, allergies, or other causes.

- Sinusitis is an inflammation and infection of the sinuses that can lead to sinus catarrh and its symptoms of facial pain, pressure, and stuffiness. Infections, allergies, and allergens are all possible sinusitis triggers.

- Catarrh can be triggered by changes in the environment, such as in temperature, humidity, and weather, especially in people with more delicate respiratory systems.

- Overconsumption of dairy products has been linked to an increase in mucus production, which in turn may cause or exacerbate catarrh in some persons.

The "milk-mucus" relationship is a common term for this, but there isn't much proof that it actually exists.

• Catarrh symptoms in patients with preexisting respiratory disorders can be exacerbated by environmental allergens such as changes in air quality, pollen levels, or the presence of specific allergens.

In order to effectively treat and manage catarrh symptoms, it is crucial to determine the root cause. It is best to see a doctor for a proper diagnosis and individualized treatment plan if catarrh persists, is severe, or is accompanied by other worrying symptoms. Depending on the source of the catarrh, treatment may involve medication, changes in lifestyle, and avoiding triggers.

CHAPTER TWO
Catarrh Symptoms

Depending on where the inflammation is and what's triggering it, catarrh can create a wide variety of symptoms. Some of the most common signs of catarrh are:

1. Symptoms of the Nose:

• Stuffy or runny nose

Constant sneezing

• Eyes that are itchy or runny (from allergies).

• A diminished or absent sense of smell or taste.

2. Tissues in the throat:

Dry coughing or coughing up mucous

Itching/irritation in the throat

• Voice alteration or hoarseness

3. Problems Breathing:

Congestion and pain in the chest.

• Breathing difficulties, most commonly associated with bronchial catarrh

Overproduction of mucus, resulting in phlegm or sputum

4. Otitis media

• A stuffed-out sensation in the ear

· Difficulty hearing (due to ear infection).

5. Chronic Sinusitis:

• Pressure and swelling around the eyes and cheekbones caused by sinus congestion

• A headache that centers on the top of the head (a sinus headache).

6. Constantly having to clean your throat

• Hack

- Feeling sick to your stomach or nauseous

Catarrh is a symptom, not a diagnosis, so it's crucial to keep that in mind. The symptoms of catarrh are most alleviated by treating the underlying problem that is causing it, which could be an infection, allergy, irritating exposure, or persistent condition.

Seek professional medical assistance if your catarrh symptoms persist or worsen, or if you have any other concerns about your health. They will be able to correctly identify your ailment, advise you on the best course of therapy, and assist you in keeping your condition under control.

The Catarrh Diagnosis

Diagnosing catarrh entails establishing the underlying cause of the excessive mucus production or inflammation in the respiratory or mucous membranes. Diagnosis is usually reached by a combination of patient history, physical exam, and other diagnostic procedures. The procedure for identifying catarrh entails the following steps:

1. Health Background:

• Your doctor will inquire about your present and previous

symptoms, how long they have lasted, and what causes or relieves them.

• Be ready to talk about any preexisting problems you have, allergies you have, irritants you've been exposed to, recent illnesses you've had, and drugs you've been prescribed.

2. Health Checkup:

• Your general health is evaluated by a physical examination, with special attention paid to the regions where catarrh has taken hold. The doctor may look in your ears, nose, and throat as well as your chest.

- They may use a lighted instrument (otoscope) to examine the ears and neck and check for symptoms of infection or inflammation.

3. Diagnosis of Symptoms:

- Your doctor will evaluate the exact catarrh symptoms you're experiencing, like a stuffy nose, cough, sore throat, or earache.

4. Diagnosing Allergies:

It may be recommended that you undergo allergy testing, such as skin prick tests or blood tests, if it is thought that allergies are the cause of your catarrh.

5. Diagnostic Imaging:

• X-rays and CT scans are two examples of imaging procedures that could be prescribed to check on the sinuses and respiratory system. Inflammation of the bronchi or sinuses can be diagnosed this way.

6. Analyses in the Lab:

• Infections or other underlying medical disorders that could be causing catarrh can be detected with laboratory testing like blood tests or cultures.

7. Nose Endoscopy: In cases of chronic nose or sinus complaints, a nasal endoscopy may be performed. A thin, flexible tube fitted with a camera (endoscope) is used to look into the nose and sinus cavities for inflammation or other problems.

8. Spirometry: Lung function tests, such as spirometry, may be performed to evaluate lung function and diagnose disorders like asthma or chronic obstructive pulmonary disease (COPD) if respiratory symptoms are present.

How you go about diagnosing what's causing your catarrh depends on your exact case. Whether it's an infection, an allergy, irritating exposure, or a persistent ailment, determining the fundamental cause allows for more effective therapy. You should see a doctor to get an accurate diagnosis and to talk about the best course of therapy for your condition.

CHAPTER THREE
Catarrh Treatment

Catarrh treatment is condition specific and should target the underlying cause. Once the doctor knows what's going on, they can prescribe medication that will help with the symptoms while also fixing the underlying problem. Some overarching strategies for dealing with catarrh are as follows:

1. Recuperate and replenish your fluids:

• To aid the body's inherent recuperative mechanisms, it is crucial to get enough sleep and drink plenty of water. Drinking plenty of fluids helps thin mucus and make it simpler to eliminate.

2. Medications:

• Symptoms of catarrh can be alleviated using over-the-counter (OTC) drugs. It's possible that these things include:

• Congestion and edema in the nasal passages can be alleviated with decongestants.

By inhibiting histamine's effects, antihistamines can be used to alleviate allergy-related congestion.

- To alleviate nighttime coughing and improve quality of sleep, cough suppressants can be helpful.

- **Expectorants:** Medications that thin and loosen mucus to facilitate coughing.

If your catarrh is severe or persistent, your doctor may prescribe medicine. Antibiotics for bacterial infections, corticosteroids for inflammation, and other treatments targeted at the underlying cause may be prescribed by your doctor.

3. Irrigating the Nose:

• Mucus buildup and stuffiness in the nose can be alleviated with the use of saline nasal rinses or sprays. These can be purchased over-the-counter or made with a simple saline solution at home.

4. Inhaling Steam:

• Steam inhalation has been shown to reduce inflammation and mucus production in the respiratory system. A steam tent can be created by placing a bowl of hot water over your head and covering yourself with a towel.

5. Gargling with Salt Water:

• Warm saltwater gargling has been shown to reduce throat irritation and pain.

6. Preventing Reactions:

• If catarrh is brought on by allergens or irritants, avoiding them might be the best course of action. Changes in behavior, such as avoiding allergens or giving up smoking, may be required.

7. Treatment of Allergies:

• Antihistamines, corticosteroids, or allergy shots, along with limiting exposure to allergens, can help with allergic catarrh.

8. Natural Cures:

• Natural remedies such as honey, ginger, and herbal teas can be helpful for some people. These remedies can help alleviate discomfort and bring about a sense of calm.

9. Treatment of Long-Term Illnesses:

• If catarrh is a symptom of a chronic condition like asthma or COPD, managing the underlying condition is key. Possible solutions include a permanent shift in diet and exercise habits.

10. Medical Operations:

• Medical or surgical procedures may be necessary in cases of chronic sinusitis or structural problems. When other treatments have failed, these may be tried.

If you want a diagnosis and treatment plan that are just right for you, you should see a doctor. Correctly identifying the source of the catarrh and treating it is essential for a successful outcome. Additionally, if catarrh is persistent, severe, or accompanied by other concerning symptoms, seeking medical advice is essential to rule out any serious underlying issues.

Catarrh Prevention

Catarrh can be difficult to avoid, but there are things you can do to lessen your chances of getting an infection or an allergic reaction. Some measures to avoid getting catarrh include:

1. Hand Washing:

Wash your hands frequently with soap and water, especially during cold and flu seasons. Prevention of viral infections that cause catarrh can be aided by regular hand washing.

2. Keep your distance:

• Keep your distance from people who are contagious if you can when they have a respiratory illness.

3. Vaccinations:

• Get the annual flu shot and any other vaccines that protect against respiratory illnesses on a regular basis.

4. Treatment of Allergies:

• Consult an allergist to determine the specific allergens that set off your catarrh and work out a treatment plan. It may involve avoiding the allergen in question, taking an antihistamine, or undergoing immunotherapy (allergy shots).

5. Clean and ventilate your home frequently to keep the air clean and healthy inside. If you have allergies, you should consider using an air purifier.

6. How to Quit Smoking:

• Please think about putting down the cigarette. Catarrh and other respiratory conditions are made more likely by the irritation caused by smoking.

7. Protect Yourself from Potentially Irritating Substances:

• Reduce your time spent in environments with potential irritants like smoke, strong odors, and chemical fumes. When working with irritants, it's important to take precautions.

8. Adequate water intake:

• Mucus can be kept thin and easier to clear if you drink plenty of water. Stay hydrated by drinking lots of water and limiting your intake of alcoholic beverages and caffeine.

9. Living a Healthy Life:

• A strong immune system and general health can be supported by following a healthy lifestyle that includes eating right and exercising regularly.

10. Adequate Procedures for Breathing:

• To avoid spreading germs when you cough or sneeze, cover your mouth and nose with a tissue or your elbow. Don't throw tissues in the trash.

11. Humidification:

• The risk of dry, irritated airways can be reduced by using a humidifier to keep humidity levels in the home at a healthy level.

12. Managing Tension:

• Chronic stress can weaken the immune system. Reduce your stress levels by doing things like yoga, meditation, and working out regularly.

13. Maintenance Checks:

• Check-ups with a doctor can help find and treat underlying health issues that could be causing your catarrh.

Even if you have a chronic condition or are allergic to a lot of things, you might not be able to completely avoid getting catarrh, but these precautions will help you avoid getting it as often and as badly. In the event that your catarrh symptoms persist or worsen, it is recommended that you see a doctor.

Catarrh is a common symptom of many respiratory issues and is therefore often associated with a wide range of conditions. **Catarrh is often accompanied by the**

following symptoms and conditions:

• Upper respiratory viral infections, such as the common cold, are a common cause of catarrh. Nasal catarrh, caused by the cold virus, can cause either a runny or stuffy nose.

• Another viral infection that can cause catarrh and its accompanying symptoms of stuffy nose, cough, and sore throat is influenza (the flu).

• Catarrh can be caused by an allergic reaction to allergens like pollen, dust, pet dander, or food. Sneezing, a runny or stuffy nose, and itchy eyes are common reactions to this.

• Congestion, facial pain, and pressure are all symptoms of sinus catarrh, which is caused by inflammation and infection of the sinuses (sinusitis).

• Acute bronchitis is often accompanied by bronchial catarrh, which is the overproduction of mucus in the bronchial tubes. Congestion of the chest and a persistent cough are common symptoms of this condition.

• Pneumonia is a more serious form of lower respiratory infection that can cause bronchial catarrh, which in turn causes a cough and breathing difficulties.

• Inflammation of the airways and increased bronchial reactivity are hallmarks of the chronic respiratory condition known as asthma. Catarrh is a common symptom of asthma, particularly during acute attacks of the disease.

• One of the two main conditions that make up COPD is chronic bronchitis, which frequently results in bronchial catarrh. COPD is characterized by chronic inflammation of the bronchi, excessive mucus production, and impaired lung function.

• Sore throat, cough, and irritation of the throat are all symptoms of throat catarrh, which can be brought on by gastroesophageal reflux disease (GERD). Reflux of stomach acid into the throat can be irritating.

• Postnasal Drip: Postnasal drip is caused by an overproduction of mucus in the nasal passages and can lead to throat catarrh and a persistent cough. This condition may result from infections, allergies, or irritants.

• Middle ear infections like otitis media can cause ear catarrh, which manifests as earache, fullness in the ear, and hearing loss.

• Catarrh symptoms in people with respiratory sensitivities can be exacerbated by environmental allergens such as changes in air quality, pollen levels, and the presence of specific allergens.

Some of the most common causes of catarrh are listed above. Understanding what's triggering your catarrh will help you find the best course of action for treating it. It is recommended to see a doctor for a diagnosis and treatment if catarrh symptoms persist or worsen, especially if you have other health concerns.

CHAPTER FOUR
Children with Catarrh

Just like in adults, there is a wide range of possible causes for catarrh in children. Finding the root of the problem is crucial for treating children with catarrh effectively. Some things to keep in mind when dealing with children's catarrh are:

1. The Same Roots:

• major colds and other viral illnesses are a major cause of catarrh in kids. Symptoms might spread from the nose and throat, causing stuffiness and runny nose.

• Catarrh can also occur in children who are allergic to pollen, dust, or animal dander, a condition known as allergic rhinitis.

Children may get catarrh if they are exposed to irritants such as secondhand smoking, harsh scents, or pollutants.

• **Sinusitis:** Infections or inflammation in the sinuses can cause sinus catarrh, leading to symptoms like sinus congestion and facial discomfort.

Common in youngsters, middle ear infections can cause ear catarrh, earache, and hearing loss.

2. Symptoms:

• Some of the symptoms of catarrh in children include: a runny or stuffy nose, coughing, sneezing, sore throat, or earache.

• Young children may not be able to verbalize their discomfort, so parents and caregivers should be aware of any changes in mood or demeanor.

3. Treatment:

• Symptom relief and treating the underlying cause are the main goals of treatment for children with catarrh.

• **Sleep:** Give the kid a good night's sleep so his or her body can heal.

• **Hydration:** Encourage youngsters to drink fluids to keep well-hydrated.

• Nasal congestion can be alleviated with OTC drugs such as saline nasal sprays or drops. Never give a youngster any medication without first talking to a doctor.

Keep kids away from smoke and other irritants in the surroundings.

If catarrh is caused by allergies, it is important to pinpoint and control those triggers. Taking allergy medicine as prescribed by a doctor is one option.

• Seek medical attention if your symptoms are severe, ongoing, or accompanied by other worrying symptoms. They are able to determine the root of the problem and offer solutions.

4. Prevention:

• To lessen the spread of infectious diseases, stress the importance of regular hand washing.

• Keep the child's living environment clean and free from potential allergens or irritants.

Vaccinate your child against diseases of the respiratory system to protect them.

In order to reduce the spread of disease, it is important to instruct older children in proper respiratory hygiene.

If you have any questions about the diagnosis, treatment, or prevention of catarrh in children, you should talk to your child's physician or other healthcare practitioner. In addition, keep an eye on kids to check on how they are doing and get them to the doctor if their symptoms get worse or if there are any worries about their health.

In the Face of Catarrh

Catarrh is annoying, but it's usually bearable if you have a plan and make some changes to your routine. The strategy to living with catarrh depends on the underlying reason and the individual symptoms experienced. Some suggestions for dealing with chronic catarrh in everyday life:

• Get to the Bottom of It If you haven't already, it's time to consult a doctor about what's causing your catarrh. You can better handle the situation and treat the underlying issue if you know what caused it.

• If your doctor has diagnosed you with a condition that causes catarrh, including allergies, asthma, or chronic sinusitis, it is important that you follow the treatment recommendations given to you. This may involve the use of drugs, alterations to one's way of life, or other methods of allergy control.

• **Keep Yourself Well-hydrated:** Thin mucus is simpler to cough up if you drink enough water throughout the day. Take in lots of fluids such as water, herbal teas, and clear broths.

• You may keep your nasal passages moist and free of excess mucus by using saline solutions, such as a nasal saline rinse or spray. When dealing with nasal catarrh, these can be extremely useful.

• Practice Good Respiratory Hygiene: To avoid the spread of illnesses or to decrease irritation, practice good respiratory hygiene by covering your mouth and nose when you cough or sneeze, and dispose of tissues correctly.

• Reduce Your Exposure to Irritants: Catarrh can be made worse by being exposed to irritants such as cigarette smoke, air pollution, harsh scents, and chemical fumes.

• Humidify the Air: Using a humidifier in your home, especially during dry or cold seasons, can assist maintain ideal humidity levels and prevent dry, irritated respiratory passages.

• If you suffer from allergies, it is important to manage environmental allergens in order to lessen the impact they have on your life. Allergy sufferers can take steps to alleviate their symptoms by reducing the amount of allergens in their environment.

• Keep an eye on what you eat: Although there isn't much evidence linking nutrition with catarrh, some people find that dairy products or specific meals might trigger or worsen mucus production. Keep an eye on what you eat for possible correlations.

• Avoiding Stress is Crucial, as it Can Worsen Catarrh Symptoms and Weaken Your Immune System. Reduce your stress levels with frequent exercise, meditation, and deep breathing exercises.

• If your catarrh lasts more than a few days, is really severe, or is accompanied by other worrying symptoms, you should see a doctor. They can determine the source of the problem and provide effective treatments.

• Always know as much as possible about your diagnosis and treatment options. The ability to make educated decisions and collaborate productively with your healthcare practitioner is facilitated by knowledge.

If you know what's causing your catarrh and take measures to alleviate your symptoms, you may find that living with it is more bearable. Have patience with yourself, and if you feel you need it, seek out professional assistance. Your doctor should be consulted for advice on how to best handle your medical condition.

Conclusion

Having catarrh means that your nose, throat, or other respiratory mucous membranes are inflamed or producing an abnormal amount of mucus. Infections, allergies, allergens, and chronic diseases are just some of the things that can set it off. The key to successful therapy and symptom management of catarrh is pinpointing its underlying etiology.

• Catarrh treatments often focus on eliminating both the underlying cause and the symptoms. These can include relaxation, hydration, over-the-counter or prescribed drugs, nasal irrigation, and lifestyle changes. Good hand cleanliness, avoiding irritants, and allergy management are all preventative strategies that can lessen the likelihood of having catarrh.

• While it's true that catarrh can make day-to-day life less than ideal, with the right treatment and lifestyle changes, most people find they can lead completely normal lives. If catarrh lasts for an extended period of time, worsens, or is accompanied by other worrying symptoms, medical attention should be sought. One's health and ability to handle catarrh can be improved by education on the condition's origins and the implementation of effective coping mechanisms.

THE END